T0144741

BASIC HEALTH PUBLICATIONS USER'S GUIDE

TO EYE HEALTH SUPPLEMENTS

Learn All about the Nutritional Supplements That Can Save Your Vision.

BILL SARDI
JACK CHALLEM Series Editor

The information contained in this book is based upon the research and personal and professional experiences of the author. It is not intended as a substitute for consulting with your physician or other healthcare provider. Any attempt to diagnose and treat an illness should be done under the direction of a healthcare professional.

The publisher does not advocate the use of any particular healthcare protocol but believes the information in this book should be available to the public. The publisher and author are not responsible for any adverse effects or consequences resulting from the use of the suggestions, preparations, or procedures discussed in this book. Should the reader have any questions concerning the appropriateness of any procedures or preparations mentioned, the author and the publisher strongly suggest consulting a professional healthcare advisor.

Series Editor: Jack Challem
Editor: Roberta W. Waddell
Typesetter: Gary A. Rosenberg
Series Cover Designer: Mike Stromberg

Basic Health Publications User's Guides are published by Basic Health Publications, Inc.

www.basichealthpub.com

ISBN: 978-1-68162-631-4

Printed in the United States of America

10   9   8   7   6   5   4   3   2   1

Contents

What Is Green Power and What Is the Best Way to Use It?

Everyone knows that eating five servings of fruits and vegetables is an important part of getting and staying healthy. Each time we're reminded that we're supposed to get our "five a day" without fail, we try anew to add these foods to our busy lives. If we find ourselves succumbing to a cold for the fifth time this winter, we promise ourselves that we'll find a way to eat better. Sometimes, even a wake-up call in the form of a severe or chronic illness may not give us sufficient motivation to eat enough fruits and vegetables on a daily basis. As easy as the health educators make it sound, getting those five servings of greens every day can be a real challenge in our fast-food-filled, stressful world.

Even if we do manage to include all of those healthy foods in our daily diets, there lies another obstacle that keeps us from achieving optimal nutrition—the ever-decreasing nutritional value of conventionally grown fruits and vegetables. Today, most fruits and vegetables are grown in depleted soil and often genetically engineered to withstand the pesticides and herbicides sprayed on them routinely. In addition, they are usually harvested well before their time to be shipped to places near and far. Conventionally raised produce tends to be much lower in essential nutrients than organically raised or homegrown varieties. However, organic food can be prohibitively expensive and difficult to obtain for the average consumer.

Fortunately, modern nutritional science enables us to create supplements that pick up where our diets leave off. This is why we recommend that you employ what we like to call "green power" to help you in your movement toward optimal health.

Green power is found in the incredible variety and quantity of vitamins, minerals, phytonutrients (plant chemicals with healing properties), enzymes, and fiber that are packed into twenty-five great greens we'll introduce you to in these pages. The best way to take advantage of green power is to use a supplement packed with these green foods, herbs, and fiber sources.

To gain its full benefits, use a powdered supplement that's cold-processed, with all of its enzymes and nutrients intact. You can add it to your everyday diet by mixing it into a glass of cold juice or water.

While not all of the great greens we'll address are actually green in color, they are all green in the sense that they come from nature, work in harmony with your body to improve your well-being, and protect you against disease.

The Top 12 Benefits of Green Power

1. Improves energy and vitality by supplying enormous amounts of concentrated vitamin and mineral nutrition.

2. Supports heart and blood vessel health by lowering "bad" LDL cholesterol levels and preventing oxidation of LDL cholesterol by free radicals—a major culprit in the artery damage that leads to heart disease.

3. Protects against type 2 diabetes by promoting blood sugar balance.

4. Greatly increases the body's antioxidant capacity so that free radicals, created by normal metabolic processes and exposure to excessive sunlight, toxins, and stress, can be neutralized before they contribute to premature aging and disease.

5. Protects against free radical attack and blood vessel clogging in the brain, thereby standing in the way of brain deterioration that can lead to foggy thinking, senility, and Alzheimer's disease.

6. Guards against liver disease by supporting the detoxification processes of the liver, improving antioxidant power in this important cleansing organ, and helping liver tissues to regenerate after damage by toxins and free radicals.

7. Protects against cancer with an array of natural substances that have been found to prevent, slow, or even reverse the growth of malignant cells.

8. Supports eye health by maintaining good circulation to the retina, which staves off age-related macular degeneration (ARMD), and by improving night vision.

9. Increases fiber intake, dramatically improving bowel function and regularity and substantially lowering risk of colon polyps and colorectal cancer.

10. Increases the number of friendly *probiotic* bacteria in your digestive, genital, and urinary tracts; these bacteria stave off less friendly bacteria and yeasts that cause infections and protect against common digestive complaints such as bloating, gas, and constipation.

11. Contains vitamins and phytonutrients that have demonstrated ability to boost immune systems function, which means improved protection against bacteria, viruses, parasites, and other pathogens (harmful foreign substances).

12. Balances and harmonizes endocrine (hormonal) function in some cases through the adaptogenic power of the great greens; optimizes your ability to handle stress, and helps your body recover from injury or illness.

25 Great Greens

1. BILBERRY (*VACCINIUM MYRTILLUS*)

Most berries pack an amazing nutritional punch. These jewel-colored, delectable fruits—particularly blueberries, cranberries, bilberries, and lingonberries, all part of the same botanical family—are chock full of vitamins and other phytonutrients that protect against disease and support a state of glowing health. The average American has never tasted bilberries, but perhaps it's time we discovered this quintessentially English fruit—especially those of us who wish we could see better in the dark.

During World War II, pilots who enjoyed jam made from bilberries as part of their daily rations reported a tremendous improvement in their night vision. Today, we know why: phytonutrients in bilberries increase eye *microcirculation* (the circulation through tiny capillaries) and regeneration of retinal purple, a substance important for night vision and good vision in general.

European bilberry is composed of about 255 *anthocyanidin pigments*—flavonoids found abundantly in deep red-blue berries. Anthocyanidins en - hance the effects of vitamin C, strengthening the walls of blood vessels throughout the body. Many eye diseases, including macular degeneration and glaucoma, arise due to the weakening of blood vessels that feed the retina and optic nerve; a daily dose of anthocyanidin-rich bilberry will help to fortify these vessels so that they can keep all the parts of the eye well-supplied with blood and nutrients. In addition, anthocyanidins and other flavonoids protect the lenses of the eyes from free radical damage that causes cataracts. Flavonoid-rich fruits also inhibit an enzyme called *aldose reductase,* which is a major cause of diabetes-related cataracts.

Flavonoids like the ones found in bilberries are also great for the lungs, protecting them against damage from secondhand smoke and other airborne pollution. They also support cardiovascular health by strengthening blood vessels throughout the body and reducing the tendency of the blood to clot excessively. Studies have shown that bilberry also protects against stroke and helps to relieve allergy symptoms. In a recent review published in the journal *Alternative Medicine Reviews,* researchers mention bilberry as part of a supplement plan useful for the management of chronic fatigue syndrome. According to another recent study, components of bilberries and other *Vaccinium* berries have anticancer activity: they stimulate the activity of enzymes that detoxify carcinogenic chemicals.

2. ACEROLA BERRY JUICE POWDER

Vitamin C was one of the first vitamins to be widely used as a nutritional supplement, thanks largely to the work of Nobel Laureate Linus Pauling. It has long been used to improve immunity, shorten the duration of colds, and foster good skin and oral health. Bright red acerola berries are nature's most abundant source of highly bioavailable vitamin C. Their juice contains ten times more vitamin C than orange juice. When they are juiced and spray-dried into powder, they provide an excellent supplemental source of this nutrient.

More than 300 biochemical reactions in the body require the participation of vitamin C, also known as *ascorbic acid.* This nutrient is an indispensable part of tissue building; without it, the body's connective tissues gradually deteriorate. Our bodies cannot make it, so it must be taken in as part of the diet. Death from the vitamin C deficiency disease, also called scurvy, was once a common plight for sailors at sea who were without fresh foods for months or years on end.

Americans spent almost $800 million on vitamin C supplements in the year 2001. A wise investment, indeed—one that protects against heart disease, vision loss, and cancer, and boosts immunity against viral and bacterial infections. It protects the skin against sun damage and supports bone and tooth health. In a study by University of California professor James E. Enstrom, people who consumed 300 to 400 mg of vitamin C daily added an extra six years to their lives!

The optimum dosage range for this nutrient varies from person to person. Those who lead high-stress lives use up vitamin C more quickly than others and may need to take higher doses. At least 500 to 1,000 mg is a good starting point; most people can take up to 10,000 mg daily without problems. Increasing your dose as soon as you begin to feel a cold or infection coming on will help you kick it sooner. If you develop diarrhea while taking a higher-than-usual dose of vitamin C, you may be taking too much; decrease the dose until the diarrhea stops.

3. ASTRAGALUS (*ASTRAGALUS MEMBRANACEOUS*)

This herb grows wild in thickets and grasslands in northwestern China, Mongolia, and Manchuria. Eastern herbalists have used the yellowish-white root of the astragalus plant for 2,000 years. It is said to support the *wei chi*, or defensive energy, of the body. Practitioners of traditional Chinese medicine (TCM) still use it to treat a wide variety of ailments, including high blood pressure, heart disease, and diabetes. By boosting immunity, this tonic herb helps to increase resistance against infectious disease and can be taken on a regular basis for this purpose. It also provides effective relief from fatigue, loss of appetite, diarrhea, and blood disorders.

Researchers at the University of Texas at Houston found that astragalus helped cancer patients with impaired immunity to regain normal immune function. Herbalists often administer astragalus to people undergoing immunity-damaging chemotherapy or radiation treatments. Children's health expert Bob Rountree, M.D., recommends astragalus as an immunity booster for children who tend to catch colds, ear infections, coughs, and sore throats often. Astragalus is a terrific general immune tonic for those who are likely to fortify themselves against these illnesses.

Other research shows that astragalus may also help to prevent the spread of malignant cancer cells into healthy tissues. In one animal study, researchers found that adding astragalus to rats' drinking water inhibited the development of mammary tumors; in a similar study, it was found that rats treated with a carcinogen plus astragalus extract were significantly less likely to develop bladder cancer than those who only got the carcinogen.

4. SPIRULINA

More than 25,000 species of algae exist on the Earth. Some are *macroalgae,* giant kelp measuring more than 150 feet long; others are microscopic single-celled *microalgae.* Micro algae evolved 3.6 billion years ago, the first photosynthetic life form to exist on the planet. They began the process of transforming carbon dioxide to oxygen that eventually allowed for the evolution of oxygen-breathing life forms like you and me.

The nutritional benefits of spirulina aren't "new" news. The Aztec Indians of Mexico used spirulina as a food source more than 500 years ago. It can be grown almost anywhere and is still a part of the diets of indigenous peoples around the world. It's a superior source of essential amino acids, essential fats, vitamins, minerals, and phytonutrients. Spirulina provides more nutrition per acre than any other food; in fact, the World Health Organization and the United Nations have both recommended spirulina as an ideal food supplement for malnourished children worldwide. Ten grams contains 460 percent of the recommended daily value (DV) for beta-carotene, 300 percent of the recommended daily value for vitamin D, 250 percent of the DV for vitamin K, and 330 percent of the DV for vitamin B_{12}. In every ten grams of spirulina, you'll also find 70 mg of calcium, 15 mg of easily absorbable iron, 40 mg of magnesium, and 140 mg of potassium. It contains all eight of the essential amino acids—those that can't be made in the body and must be taken in through the diet.

Spirulina evolved without a rigid cell wall, and thus is very easily broken down, absorbed, and assimilated, even by those with poor digestion. It's highly alkaline, with a pH of 8—an excellent way to balance the acidity of a diet rich in acid-producing foods such as meats and dairy products. As the foods we eat become more and more drained of nutrients due to depleted soil and modern, chemical-friendly farming techniques, spirulina supplementation may well become a vital way to put nutrition back into the food supply. As it is, spirulina is already being used to fortify the nutrient-poor diets of livestock, decreasing the need to dose them up with antibiotics.

Spirulina is one of nature's best sources of gamma-linoleic acid (GLA), an omega-6 fatty acid that's lacking in the average meat-rich, processed-food diet. GLA is an important component of breast milk, and is also found in evening primrose, borage, and blackcurrant oils. Supplemental GLA has been found to help ease autoimmune inflammatory conditions such as rheumatoid arthritis, as well as PMS and skin conditions.

Substances found abundantly in this microalgae also support intestinal production of friendly bacteria and suppress the growth of unfriendly *candida* yeasts and *E. coli* bacteria.

Research into the benefits of spirulina as a dietary supplement has exploded over the past thirty years. Studies have shown that it has beneficial effects on immune system function, increasing the body's production of immune cells (*antibodies* and *cytokines*) and boosting the ability of T and B cells to fend off bacteria and viruses. This makes spirulina an excellent choice for people whose immune systems are compromised, especially those who are undergoing radiation or chemotherapy treatments for cancer. One test-tube study examined immune system activation by polysaccharides (carbohydrates) isolated from spirulina. Researchers found that the spirulina polysaccharides activated certain immune cells 100 to 1,000 times better than the medications currently given to cancer patients to boost their immunity. Cancer patients undergoing radiation are vulnerable to bone marrow damage—bone marrow is where many immune cells are made—

and research has shown that spirulina protects bone marrow against the ravages of radiation therapy.

With its bounty of the cleansing green pigment chlorophyll and other liver-supporting nutrients, spirulina has been shown to protect against liver disease. It prevents the formation of damaged liver tissues in diabetic animals and improves the condition of human subjects with chronic liver disease. Spirulina is also protective against lead poisoning, helping the body to get rid of excess lead and buffering the free radical explosion that causes the ill effects of lead poisoning. Other research supports its anti-inflammatory and antioxidant effects; it contains a newly discovered antioxidant called *phycocyanin,* a blue-green pigment that is thought to be spirulina's main antioxidant-boosting component. Phycocyanin, alpha-carotene, beta-carotene, gamma-carotene, and xanthophylls all work together to improve antioxidant power. These and other substances found in spirulina have been found to be active against the herpes virus, AIDS, cytomegalovirus, and the flu virus.

Spirulina also has cancer-preventative effects. It appears to be especially effective against mouth cancer. In one study, the use of only one gram of spirulina a day brought about complete regression of oral cancer lesions in 44 percent of the male tobacco chewers who participated.

Spirulina has been shown to protect the body against the adverse effects of toxic chemicals. We're surrounded by such chemicals, and while it's a good idea to do what you can to avoid exposure, you also need to supply your body with the functional foods that will help it to cleanse itself of these toxins. In one study, one group of rats was given either spirulina or chlorella (a green food we'll discuss later in this book) while another group was given a regular diet of rat chow; both groups were also given doses of the dangerous chemical dioxin. The rats consuming spirulina or chlorella were able to eliminate *seven times* the amount of dioxin compared to the rats who got none of these green foods. In another study, mice given spirulina before being given carcinogenic chemicals showed significantly less damage to their DNA and lower levels of free radical activity than their non-spirulina-eating counterparts.

5. GRAPE SEED EXTRACT

In 1966, Jacques Masquelier, Ph.D., and his research team at the University of Bordeaux in France, rediscovered a cold remedy that had been used 400 years earlier by North American Indians as a treatment for scurvy, the vitamin C deficiency disease. Derived from the bark of French maritime pine trees, Dr. Masquelier's discovery was a unique type of bioflavonoid nutrient, known today as the *oligomeric proanthocyanidins* (OPCs). The OPCs in maritime pines—usually sold under the trade name Pycnogenol—turned out to be identical in chemical structure to those found in the seeds and skins of red and purple grapes and in the deeply hued wines made from these grapes. Grape seed extract (GSE) is now thought to be a superior source of these OPCs, and most of the research on OPCs has been conducted with GSE rather than Pycnogenol.

Today, we know that these OPCs are one of the most important reasons that people who indulge moderately in red wine tend to be healthier and live longer. Even if you do enjoy a glass of red wine now and then, you can get additional OPCs directly from the most abundant source (grape seeds are 95 percent OPCs) by supplementing your diet with grape seed extract.

OPCs are twenty times more potent than vitamin C and fifty times more potent than vitamin E when it comes to protecting the body against the ravages of free radicals. In addition, they have the ability to quickly replenish spent vitamin C, as well as vitamin E. GSE and maritime pine bark extract work as treatments for scurvy not only because they contain vitamin C; the OPCs that they contain have the ability to "rejuvenate" spent vitamin C, making better use of what is available. OPCs have another advantage over other antioxidants: they easily pass through the blood-brain barrier into brain tissues, which many nutrients can't do. As a result, OPCs, like GSE, protect the brain against free radical attack—one of the established causes of Alzheimer's disease.

Studies have shown that OPCs improve the strength of capillary walls, making them an effective preventative against varicose veins, leg swelling, and *retinopathy* (deterioration of the eye's retina due to "leaky" capillaries). Their general strengthening effect on blood vessel walls and the function of the cardiovascular system makes OPCs a good addition to any heart disease prevention program. They have been found to inhibit lipid peroxidation, or free radical attack on "bad" LDL cholesterol—a process that greatly increases the danger these fats pose to blood vessel walls. OPCs also protect against cardiovascular disease by decreasing the tendency of blood to clot. In fact, the OPCs found in red wine are thought to explain the so-called "French Paradox"—the fact that the French, despite their diet full of rich foods, have far lower heart disease rates than those in the United States.

Skin aging and loss of skin elasticity can be curbed with the circulation-stimulating effects of GSE. Other research indicates that asthma, allergies, and severe inflammation can be eased with GSE, and that GSE has antibacterial and antiviral effects that support immunity against infectious diseases.

One study found that liver, lung, and heart toxicity caused by overdoses of prescription drugs were reduced when test animals were given GSE before drug administration. Still more research demonstrates that GSE is protective against stress-induced ulcers. This type of ulcer is caused by high levels of an inflammatory substance called histamine, and GSE binds to the stomach lining and protects it against its erosive effects.

6. ROYAL JELLY

The queen bee is born to humble beginnings. She hatches from the exact same eggs as her worker-bee siblings. Although she is genetically identical to her sisters, she grows 40 to 60 percent larger than they do, and she spends her life producing two and a half times her own body weight in eggs every single day. Despite her heavy workload, the queen bee lives four to five times longer than worker bees do. How does she do it? Apparently, it has much to do with the fact that she is fed on a steady diet of royal jelly from the day she is born.

Milky white royal jelly is secreted by worker bees specifically for the nourishment of newly hatched members of the swarm, but the queen bee is the only one who dines exclusively on this nutrient-rich superfood. Royal jelly contains a full storehouse of B vitamins, including B_1, B_2, biotin, folic acid, and B_{12}; it is an especially good source of pantothenic acid (B_5), a B vitamin known to help the body cope better with stress. A full complement of amino acids, including the eight essential amino acids, can also be found in royal jelly, which is approximately 12 percent protein. Royal jelly also contains small amounts of several essential minerals, including calcium, copper, iron, phosphorus, potassium, silicon, and sulfur.

In addition, royal jelly contains fatty acids, including a little-understood compound known as *10-hydroxy-2-decanoic acid* (10-HDA). Early research shows that this compound could be the substance responsible for the queen bee's size and incredible fertility. Studies by Japanese scientists have revealed that 10-HDA also may have antibacterial properties, and research is underway to explore potential uses of 10-HDA as a cancer preventative. Athletes who use royal jelly report that their stamina improves. Research shows that royal jelly may have cholesterol-lowering effects and that it speeds the healing of skin wounds. Substances contained in royal jelly have been found to resist bacteria and viruses. In the digestive tract, components of royal jelly are transformed into a natural blood-pressure-lowering substance. Studies have shown that royal jelly supplementation can lower blood cholesterol levels significantly and that it decreases the tendency of blood to form dangerous clots.

A word of caution to asthmatics and those with eczema or allergies:

royal jelly does contain pollen and has very rarely been linked to severe allergic reactions. If, within a few minutes to several hours after you take royal jelly, you experience a runny nose, itchy, puffy eyes, rash, hives, wheezing, or shortness of breath, you may be having an allergic reaction. If this happens to you, seek medical attention right away. It should also be noted, however, that Japanese research has shown that royal jelly actually has anti-allergy effects, sometimes slowing the processes that cause allergic-inflammations.

Use a product that contains freeze-dried, powdered royal jelly. This delicate food doesn't keep well unless it's either preserved in honey or freeze-dried soon after harvesting.

7. LICORICE ROOT EXTRACT

When you think of licorice, you probably think of red or black candy ropes packaged in plastic. This type of candy was once flavored with real licorice root, but today it bears resemblance to the herb in nothing other than its name. An entirely different plant, anise, is actually the source of modern licorice candy's distinctive flavor.

Licorice is a perennial plant that grows wild in parts of Asia and in southern and central Europe. Today, it is also cultivated in the United States and Canada. Licorice root has a long history of medicinal use, dating back thousands of years. It is one of the top five medicinal herbs used by practitioners of traditional Chinese medicine (TCM), often incorporated into herbal formulas to harmonize other ingredients. Its root contains both its medicinal ingredients and *glycyrrhizin,* a substance that is roughly fifty times sweeter than sugar cane.

Licorice root, when chewed or sucked on, helps to increase saliva and mucus flow, and softens, soothes, nourishes, and lubricates the gastrointestinal tract. It's a great remedy for heartburn, acid reflux, and ulcers because it actually coats and protects the esophagus, stomach, and intestines. Licorice also has a mild stimulating effect on the adrenal gland. These glands make *cortisol,* an important anti-inflammatory, energizing hormone. As a result of this gentle stimulation, licorice helps boost energy and vitality.

Licorice root also shows promise as an anticancer agent. It ranks among the most potent cancer-protective plants, on par with garlic, soy, cabbage, and ginger. Many studies have shown that licorice root extracts may protect against the DNA damage caused by carcinogens—the initial insult that leads to cancer formation—and that they may also suppress the growth of cancers that have already formed. The most promising results have been found in breast and prostate cancer studies.

Research has shown that licorice is an effective antiviral and antibacterial agent. It also works as an anti-inflammatory, which explains its soothing effects on mucous membranes throughout the body, including those in the nasal passages and bronchial tubes. Both of these airways can become uncomfortably inflamed in people with chronic allergies or asthma.

Licorice also has phytoestrogenic effects. It contains substances that act like mild estrogens in the body, blocking the carcinogenic effects of estrogenic chemicals (*xenoestrogens*), which are impossible to avoid in the modern world. Both men and women will benefit from this xenoestrogen-blocking effect of licorice root.

If you have high blood pressure, you should be aware that licorice root can exacerbate this problem in some people. When you first add this herb to your supplement regimen, keep track of your blood pressure. If it rises to undesirable levels in response to the herb, you may want to try lowering the dose or using *deglycyrrhizinated* licorice extract (DGL), from which the blood-pressure-raising glycyrrhizin has been removed.

8. SIBERIAN GINSENG (*ELEUTHEROCOCCUS SENTICOSUS*)

Siberian ginseng is one of the best-known adaptogenic herbs. Adaptogens are herbs that improve the body's overall state of balance and support its ability to resist the detrimental effects of stress. Known to many as the "king of adaptogens," Siberian ginseng was discovered by Russian scientist I. I. Brekhman, M.D., Ph.D. He traveled throughout Siberia, asking the people who lived and worked there how they managed to keep their strength and energy up through the long winters. They attributed much of their hardiness to the plant that is known today as Siberian ginseng. While not a true member of the ginseng plant family, this herb is so-named because its effects are very similar to those other ginsengs.

In studies of tens of thousands of Soviet factory workers, Olympic athletes, and astronauts, researchers found that those individuals who regularly took Siberian ginseng were more productive and had improved stamina. The longer the herb was taken, the more pronounced its effects proved to be. Since that time, further studies have shown that Siberian ginseng facilitates adaptation to a wide variety of stressful circumstances, including extremes of temperature, injury recovery, jet lag, immobilization, and high-dose hormone therapy.

Research has shown that Siberian ginseng enhances the function of the endocrine system, the system of glands and hormones that orchestrates so many of the body's day-to-day functions. Amazingly, it has the ability to both boost the production of hormones that are low and decrease the production of hormones that are being overproduced. By regulating the way in which sugars are stored and released into the bloodstream, Siberian ginseng helps to maintain steady blood sugar balance. It also has antiviral and anti-allergy activity, improves immune function and mental clarity, normalizes blood pressure, reduces fatigue, and relieves depression.

9. SUMA (*PFAFFIA PANICULATA*)

Suma—also known as Brazilian ginseng—is a large ground vine that grows wild in South America. It has been used as an herbal tonic, energizer, rejuvenator, and aphrodisiac in South America for more than 300 years. Today, it remains an important remedy for a wide variety of ailments in indigenous Indian populations. European herbalists use suma to strengthen immune function, treat infertility, and stimulate and balance the function of the endocrine system. Russian athletes use it to build endurance and muscle. With all of these uses, it's no wonder that in Portuguese suma is referred to as *para todo,* meaning "for everything."

Suma is an adaptogenic herb that has been shown to have tremendous capacity for building up the immune system. Japanese researchers, often at the forefront when it comes to new discoveries about herbal medicine, have isolated phytochemicals from suma called *pfaffosides* that inhibit tumor cell growth. A compound called *allantoin* is also found in suma; this substance is known to promote the growth of healthy new cells and the healing of wounds.

Other research has revealed that suma phytosterols, such as *beta-ecdysone,* have hormone like effects in the body, enhancing protein synthesis and helping to improve physical endurance. By stimulating this and other *anabolic* (rebuilding) processes, suma aids in tissue repair and strengthening. *Sitosterol* and *stigmasterol* are other phytosterols found in suma, and they lend support to the body by nourishing the circulatory and endocrine (glandular) systems. Their hormonelike effects could explain why many herbalists use suma to treat menopausal and menstrual symptoms. Sitosterol and stigmasterol have been found to be beneficial for circulatory health, improving circulation to the muscular walls of the heart and balancing blood cholesterol levels. In addition, it is also said that suma helps to enhance sexual function.

A rare mineral salt called germanium is also found in suma. Germanium promotes optimal oxygen flow to the cells. Iron, phosphorus, potassium, copper, calcium, vitamins A, B_1, B_2, C, D, E, and K, and several amino acids are part of suma's nutrient bounty. You can benefit from suma if you're simply looking for a boost, or if you suffer from chronic stress, high blood pressure, anemia, liver disease, chronic viral infections, diabetes, poor digestion, or skin problems.

10. NOVA SCOTIA DULSE (*RHODYMENIA PALMATA*)

Dulse is a variety of ocean plants similar to kelp. It grows in the mid-tide portion of the intertidal zone, which is why you'll often see this reddish-purple, 16- to 18-inch long sea plant lying exposed to the air during low tide. It has served as a concentrated source of nutrients and as a delicious flavoring agent in many cuisines since antiquity, but Westerners are only just beginning to rediscover it.

Unlike foods grown in depleted soil, dulse is loaded with trace minerals that the body can easily utilize. It is an excellent source of the mineral iodine, which is necessary for good thyroid function. Until the widespread use of iodized salt, iodine deficiency caused many cases of underactive thyroid (hypothyroidism) and goiter—a swelling of the thyroid that signifies advanced hypothyroidism—in parts of the world far from the seas.

Dulse harvested off the coast of Nova Scotia is darker and thicker than dulse harvested elsewhere. Due to the ideal growing environment of the region, the plant concentrates more nutrients into its leaves, which translates to a better source of supplemental nutrients. If you like the taste of dulse, you can buy it in an Asian or health food market, lightly toast it, grind it up, and sprinkle it over foods as you would any condiment. You can also take powdered dulse in supplemental form.

11. CHLORELLA

Since the Precambrian era more than 2.5 billion years ago, this one-celled freshwater algae has lived on the Earth. In fact, chlorella was the first form of cell to develop a true nucleus. Chlorella is surrounded by a strong cell wall—so strong, in fact, that chlorella with an intact cell wall is significantly more difficult to digest and assimilate than chlorella that has been treated (without heat) to break up the cell's wall.

Chlorella can very effectively repair its genetic material, or DNA. This enables it to reproduce itself perfectly and rapidly. In an ideal environment, it quadruples itself in only seventeen to twenty hours time! This characteristic makes nutrient-dense chlorella an ideal food source in third world nations; it can be grown rapidly and without much care.

Chlorella contains nearly twice the protein of soybeans and eight times that of rice. It's loaded with more than twenty vitamins and minerals and the nucleic acids DNA and RNA, as well as the important omega-3 and omega-6 fats. It also contains more of the bright green pigment chlorophyll than any other known plant—hence the name, *chlorella*. Chlorophyll is one of the most health-supporting components of this green food.

Chlorella's list of benefits is a startlingly long one. Research has shown that it effectively scavenges free radicals. It detoxifies the body of heavy metal, pesticides, and other highly toxic chemicals—all of which have been linked with increased risk of cancer, heart disease, and liver disease—by binding to these substance in the body. In Japan, where 1,000 tons of chlorella are produced each year, residents use it regularly to protect themselves against the ill effects of radiation and air pollution.

Chlorella improves the ability of the liver to detoxify the body. One of the best illustrations of this, aside from its protective effects against toxic chemicals and heavy metals, is that certain studies have shown taking 4 to 5 grams before a night of drinking can completely prevent a hangover the following day! It also fosters increased production of "good" lactobacillus and vitamin B_{12}—forming bacteria in the gastrointestinal tract.

Immune function—in particular, that of the macrophages, which attack and engulf bacteria and cancer cells—is increased by chlorella. When given chlorella, animals with tumors lived longer because of this increased macrophage activity. Chlorella is high in beta-carotene, which kills cancer cells. It protects heart health by lowering high blood pressure, and appears to inhibit the thickening of the arterial wall that leads to narrowed blood vessels and heart attacks.

Chlorella serves to detoxify the bowels and quickly relieves bad breath, chronic constipation, and intestinal gas. Some research indicates that it may be an effective treatment for ulcers. Applying chlorella to areas of skin that have been injured or that have been affected by dermatitis has been found to speed healing, and some users report that taking it by mouth has been an effective treatment for acne. Fatigue, asthma, and allergies are other maladies that have reportedly been helped with chlorella supplementation.

Don't expect results immediately with chlorella. Like any natural substance, it tends to work slowly over a period of months. Some people, however, do feel a difference as soon as they begin to use it!

12. APPLE PECTIN

Since the nineteenth century campaign on behalf of whole-grain foods by graham cracker inventor Sylvester Graham, followed soon after by appeals to add roughage to the diet from breakfast cereal entrepreneur John Harvey

Kellogg, the health benefits of whole grains and bran have been a topic of much discussion in the Western, white-bread-loving world. At one time, it was thought that the removal of fiber would make foods more nutritious.

Today—now that we've grown accustomed to the light texture and sweet taste of refined grains—we're paying the price for messing with Mother Nature. Constipation, hemorrhoids, colon cancer, diverticulosis/ diverticulitis, blood sugar imbalance, and a host of other complaints can be traced, at least in part, back to the lack of whole grains, fruits and vegetables, and the fiber they contain. If you've been eating the largely fiber*less* Standard American Diet (SAD) for most of your lifetime, adding supplemental fiber to your diet in the form of apple pectin is a good step to take.

Pectins are soluble fibers, meaning that they are transformed into a gel when they come in contact with water. While insoluble fibers improve health by increasing the bulk and water content of bowel movements, soluble fibers do so by stabilizing blood sugar, reducing cholesterol and blood pressure, and providing an ideal environment for the growth of friendly colon bacteria (such as *lactobacillus* and *bifiduc*). These friendly bacteria are your allies when it comes to digestive health, protecting the gastrointestinal (GI) tract against less friendly bacteria, yeast overgrowth, and carcinogens.

Apple pectin is one of the reasons that an apple a day keeps the doctor away. In one study by the John Hopkins Medical Institute, a bowl of oatmeal or buckwheat a day—like apple pectin, both excellent sources of soluble fiber —lowered cholesterol and blood pressure levels. Soluble fiber slows the absorption of sugar through the intestinal walls and into the bloodstream, which explains its balancing effects on blood sugar. Apple pectin is a particularly good supplement for those with chronically high blood sugar or type 2 diabetes. Not only does it help to control blood glucose levels, it controls other risk factors for heart disease, which type 2 diabetics are especially prone to. Apple pectin has been shown time and again to significantly lower "bad" LDL cholesterol without lowering "good" HDL cholesterol.

In a recently published study, mice with a genetic predisposition for colon cancer were treated with a carcinogenic chemical. A combination of apple pectin *Bifidobacterium longum* bacteria reduced both the number and severity of colon tumors in these mice. Another study showed that apple pectin had an anti-inflammatory effect on the GI tract—an important point in light of recent discoveries about the role of inflammation in colon cancer—and significantly decreased the likelihood that colon tumors would spread to the livers of lab animals.

A Ukrainian study illustrated that apple pectin binds to some toxic heavy metals and draws them out of the body before they can be absorbed. Other research shows that apple pectin has a bacteriostatic effect, meaning that it slows or stops the activity of unfriendly bacteria. In a study by Russian researchers, some patients hospitalized with gastrointestinal infections were given supplemental apple pectin, while others received only the typical antibiotic treatment for their illnesses. Patients who were given apple pectin left the hospital an average of two to three days sooner.

13. BROWN RICE GERM

For two-thirds of the world's population, rice is an irreplaceable part of each day's meals. When first harvested from the paddy, rice kernels are encased in an inedible husk, which is removed to reveal brown rice. To make white rice—the kind of rice normally eaten by Westerners—the bran and germ must also be removed. While white, "polished" rice cooks more quickly and agrees with the taste buds, it has also been stripped of its vitamins, minerals, and fiber.

If you've been eating white rice all of your life, try to add some brown rice to your diet. It has a nutty, wholesome taste that white rice just can't match, although it might take some getting used to. Also consider adding extra insoluble fiber to your supplement plan with brown rice germ. Unlike soluble fiber, insoluble fibers don't change when water is added. When you think of fiber as a "broom" that sweeps your GI tract clean, you're thinking of the insoluble variety. When you're taking in adequate fiber—at least 30 grams a day is optimal—and enough water, your bowel movements will be more regular. In parts of the world where whole foods are staples and diets are naturally high in fiber, the amount of time it takes for the remnants of a meal to pass out of the body (transit time) is only about twenty-four hours on average. That means that any putrefactive bacteria, extra hormones, carcinogens, or other toxic substances don't hang around in the colon for long before they're eliminated. When transit time stretches to two or three days, as is common in places where processed, fiberless foods are the norm, all of these toxins sit in the colon. Here, they brew additional toxins that may be absorbed back into the body, potentially causing changes in the colon that could someday lead to colon cancer.

An additional benefit of using rice germ: research has shown that the nutritious parts of brown rice—in other words, the bran and germ—contain *phenols,* substances that inhibit the growth of human breast and colon cancer cells. The oils found in the husks of brown rice also have healing properties; studies have demonstrated that these oils have the power to lower high cholesterol levels.

14. GREEN TEA EXTRACT

In this nation of coffee drinkers, tea drinkers have a leg up when it comes to having a long and healthy life. The medicinal benefits of tea have been widely known since the year 1211, when Eisai Myoan—the Japanese founder of the modern-day Zen Buddhism movement—wrote the first book on the subject. Green tea, a variety of tea made with leaves that have undergone less processing than those in black varieties, is typically consumed in Asian nations. Until recently, green tea had been virtually unheard of in the West. Now that its health-supporting qualities are gaining recognition worldwide, green tea is growing in popularity in Western nations as well.

Much of the research into green tea's health benefits concern a phytochemical called *epigallocatechin gallate* (EGCG). Carcinogens often damage DNA by creating intense bursts of reactive free radicals; EGCG neutralizes free radicals at an amazing rate, protecting cells against the damage they can do. In fact, one recent study showed that green tea offers 200 times more antioxidant protection than vitamin E! This helps to explain its protective effects against both cancer and heart disease. Cancer often starts out with free radical damage to DNA, which studies have shown time and again is prevented even by low concentrations of EGCG. When free radicals attack LDL cholesterol in the bloodstream, it becomes *oxidized* and far more harmful to blood vessel walls; EGCG inhibits this process of LDL oxidation.

Epigallocatechin gallate is one of several green tea polyphenols, powerful antioxidants that protect cells against free radical assault. These polyphenols have been shown to inhibit the growth of tumors by several mechanisms: they activate enzymes that detoxify the body of carcinogens; they put the brakes on the process of angiogenesis, where tumors grow blood vessels that allow them to become larger; they inhibit the expression of a gene that promotes cancer, as well as chronic inflammatory diseases such as rheumatoid arthritis and multiple sclerosis; they slow the multiplication of cancer cells and encouraging apoptosis, or cell death. (Apoptosis is actually a good thing when it comes to cancer. Cancer is basically the uncontrolled multiplication of cells that don't die and don't do anything but use up nutrients and take up space.) EGCG also inhibits the formation of *urokinase,* an enzyme critical to cancer growth.

Several studies show that green tea extracts offer excellent protection against skin cancer. The formation of nitrosamines—carcinogenic byproducts of chemicals used in meat processing and a major cause of stomach cancer—is also blocked by green tea polyphenols. Cancer researchers have discovered that *theanine,* a unique amino acid that gives green tea its taste, enhances the effectiveness of several cancer medications and reduces their side effects. If you are fighting cancer, be sure to add green tea to your daily regimen, especially before, during, and after chemotherapy and radiation.

Green tea has antiviral and antibacterial effects and helps to promote better digestion, increasing the population of friendly bacteria and decreasing that of less beneficial ones. It also protects against gum disease by killing plaque and bacteria in the mouth.

15. BRAN

Bran—whether derived from rice or wheat—is an excellent supplemental source of soluble fiber. Several studies have shown that diets high in bran reduce the risk of developing colon polyps (a precancerous condition) and colon cancer. One such study, from Cornell Medical Center, showed that colon polyps shrank in subjects who ate high-fiber wheat bran cereal for four years.

One study demonstrated that a diet supplement with wheat bran caused changes in the activity of enzymes that neutralize and get rid of *xenobiotic* chemicals. Xenobiotics are synthetic substances with structural similarities to estrogen; when they enter the body, they behave like estrogens with attitudes, potentially causing changes that will lead to cancer.

Excess estrogens are disposed of via the gastrointestinal tract. While they sit in the colon, these estrogens are altered into more active—and therefore, more carcinogenic—forms. If they aren't eliminated quickly, they seep back into the body through the colon wall.

Both soluble and insoluble fibers increase the feelings of satiety, causing you to feel full sooner during a meal. Adding a fiber supplement to your diets could help you to eat less and lose weight.

16. SPROUTED BARLEY MALT

Sprouts are one of nature's most energizing superfoods. When a seed, whole grain, or legume is just beginning to sprout into a mature plant, it has all the nutritional characteristics of the highly nutritious whole food plus those of a vegetable at its most nutrient-dense, enzyme-rich stage. Sprouted barley malt is a source of soluble fiber derived from this delicious sprout. It has a pleasantly sweet taste and serves as a food source for the friendly bacteria in the digestive tract. Using supplemental barley malt to add to your fiber intake will help relieve constipation, irritable bowel syndrome, and diverticulosis. Its balancing effects on blood sugar will help to protect you against type 2 diabetes and chronic blood sugar leaps and dips.

17. NATURAL CHLOROPHYLL

Chlorophyll is, in essence, plant blood. It's startlingly similar in molecular structure to the hemoglobin molecule, which is responsible for carrying oxygen in the bloodstream of humans and animals. The pH of chlorophyll is 7.4, exactly that of human blood. The only difference is that magnesium is at chlorophyll's core, while iron is at the core of hemoglobin.

Chlorophyll is created when sunshine strikes the surfaces of plants. Liquid chlorophyll, extracted from healthy, bright green flora, has been used by natural healers for years. It has a cleansing, deodorizing effect on the gastrointestinal tract, making it a wonderful remedy for chronic bad breath. As a mouth rinse, chlorophyll is useful for healing oral diseases such as tooth decay and pyorrhea. Many midwives advise their pregnant patients to drink water with chlorophyll added, or "green water," to build the strength of their blood and assist their livers in disposing of toxins throughout their pregnancies. Chlorophyll is an excellent source of minerals, vitamins, and trace elements. Natural healers have also reported success in treating kidney stones and upper respiratory infections with the help of this green elixir.

Chlorophyll may help support immunity against the spread of cancer cells and other *pathogens* (harmful organisms). Cancer cells and other path - ogens manufacture specialized enzymes to break down the membranes of adjoining cells; this allows them to spread easily. Chlorophyll has been found to ward off the actions of those enzymes, thereby protecting healthy cells against invasion.

18. DAIRY-FREE PROBIOTIC CULTURE

In the Middle East, milk fermented with bacteria has been used to treat and prevent illness for centuries. In the early 1900s, Nobel Prize-winning scientist Elie Metchnikoff showed that this benign bacteria—called *lacto - bacillus*—transformed the lactose in milk into lactic acid. This process gave the milk a sour taste, greater digestibility, a thickened texture, and resistance to disease-producing bacteria. Today, we know milk with lactobacillus culture added as yogurt. Dr. Metchnikoff knew that there was something special about this dynamic combination of milk and bacteria, having found that Bulgarians who made fermented buttermilk a dietary staple enjoyed life spans significantly longer than average. Research has continued to show that yogurt supports good health, and this is largely due to the lactobacilli and other *probiotic* bacteria it contains.

Daily intake of probiotics controls the growth of toxin-producing putrefactive bacteria in the gastrointestinal tract. Probiotics beat out "bad" bacteria in several ways: if the population of good bacteria is high, they crowd out the bad; they create an acidic environment that is not supportive of growth of bad bacteria; and they produce antibiotic-like substances called *bacteriocins.*

Probiotic bacteria manufacture several different B vitamins, which can then be absorbed into the bloodstream through the intestinal walls. They also improve digestion by helping to break down proteins, fats, and carbohydrates. Probiotics don't just live in the digestive tract; they also populate the urinary tract, genital tract, and skin. They are instrumental in warding off yeasts, fungi, and bacteria that can cause infections. Supplemental probiotics are especially effective at preventing vaginal infections. Probiotics maintain vaginal pH in a range that isn't conducive to the growth of harmful yeasts or trichomonas bacteria.

The benefits of probiotics are far-reaching. Studies have shown that the nutrients contained in foods fermented with probiotics are more easily assimilated. Studies of both humans and animals show that lactobacillus supplementation effectively lowers cholesterol levels; other studies indicate that foods and supplements containing these friendly bacteria inhibit the growth of cancerous tumors, enhance immunity, and are useful for the treatment and prevention of constipation, diarrhea, and food poisoning.

Probiotics are important detoxifiers that rid the body of carcinogenic substances. For example, research has shown that high numbers of unfriendly bacteria in the colon (including campylobacter, *E. coli,* clostridium, and streptococcus) indicate an increased risk of developing colon cancer. These bacteria manufacture toxins that threaten the health of the intestines and—if they are absorbed through the intestinal wall—the entire body. In a study published in the *Asian Medical Journal,* supplementation with large doses of live lactobacilli significantly lowered the activity of these unfriendly bacteria.

While small amounts of unsweetened, minimally processed fermented milk products such as yogurt are healthful additions to your diet, most of us will need a little extra help in the form of a probiotic supplement. Choose a dairy-free, freeze-dried probiotic version. And always be sure to use a probiotic supplement as soon as you finish a course of antibiotics, because prescription antibiotics will dramatically cut down on the number of probiotic bacteria in your body. Ideally, you should use a supplement that contains 2.5 billion lactobacilli per dose.

19. MILK THISTLE (*SILYBUM MARIANUM*) EXTRACT

Also known as St. Mary's Thistle and Our Lady's Thistle, milk thistle can grow to be more than six feet tall. Its coarse, prickly-edged leaves are lined with white veins, which release a milky juice when crushed—hence, the herb's more popular name.

Milk thistle has been used to support liver health for almost 2,000 years. Today, it is a well-known natural treatment for cirrhosis of the liver, fatty liver, and chronic hepatitis. This herb isn't just for people who already have liver disease, however. In the modern world, our livers are forced to work overtime processing toxins from pollution, processed foods, hormone-mimicking chemicals, and medications. Using milk thistle to shore up this important cleansing organ against everyday stresses will go a long way toward preventing liver disease in the future.

Liver health is underappreciated in Western medicine. Eastern forms of medicine, such as traditional Chinese medicine and Ayurveda, emphasize that if the liver and other cleansing organs aren't in good working order, the health of the entire body is adversely affected. The effectiveness of milk thistle in treating skin conditions is an excellent illustration of this principle.

Within the seeds of milk thistle lies a bioflavonoid complex called *silymarin*. Silymarin has antioxidant power many times that of vitamin E, and for reasons we don't quite understand, it zeros in on the liver. It protects the liver against free radicals naturally formed in the detoxification process, and boosts levels of antioxidant enzymes such as *glutathione* and *superoxide dismutase* in the liver. Milk thistle increases the regeneration of liver cells by an astonishing 400 to 500 percent. In addition, this ancient herb decreases harmful inflammation. Another of the phytochemicals found in milk thistle, *silibinin* has been found to inhibit the growth of several different kinds of cancer cells, including cancer of the prostate. Taking 200 mg three times a day will do much to keep your liver—and the rest of you—in a state of glowing good health.

20. ECHINACEA

The purple coneflower plant, commonly known as echinacea, has been used for centuries by Plains Indians for the treatment of bites, coughs, sore throats, toothaches, and infections. This member of the daisy family had healing properties impressive enough that the first American settlers began to use it as well, and sent word back to Europe about this powerful herbal remedy. Until after the end of World War II, echinacea continued to be a popular home remedy; but it was soon forgotten as antibiotic drugs became widely available. The Germans continued to use and study echinacea, and today it is reemerging as one of the most thoroughly researched and widely used herbs in the world.

Study after study has illustrated echinacea's effectiveness in boosting immune function. The process of *phagocytosis*—where white blood cells surround, engulf, and destroy pathogens—is measurably enhanced by echinacea extract. Echinacea also enhances immune cells' ability to "zap" pathogens with powerful free radicals called the *superoxide anion*. (While free radicals can cause serious harm when they're overproduced, immune cells actually use them as weapons against foreign invaders!) Dozens of published studies have demonstrated that echinacea helps people get well faster when they're stricken with colds, flus, or other infections. Other research indicates that echinacea protects against infections by inhibiting the formation of *hyaluronidase* enzyme—an enzyme that eats away the natural barriers set up by healthy cells against pathogens.

21. ALFALFA

Many of the sprouts you find packaged in your supermarket are grown from tiny alfalfa seeds. When you eat sprouted seeds, you're capturing them at a very special time in their growth—when they're packed with the energy, enzymes, and nutrients that, in nature, the sprout would need to take root and develop into a mature plant. Alfalfa is a good source of vitamin K, which supports healthy blood clotting, helps to prevent hemorrhages, and aids in the retention of that all-important mineral, calcium.

One study of alfalfa supplementation showed that this humble plant can cut harmful LDL cholesterol levels. This translates to added protection against coronary artery disease and stroke.

22. BARLEY

Have you ever sat down to a steaming hot bowl of homemade beef barley soup? If so, you satisfied more than your taste buds by eating a helping of this wonderful grain. You also helped to satisfy your body's need for soluble fiber. Barley is an excellent source of soluble fiber, just like apple pectin. A study from Montana State University showed that subjects who ate a barley-rich diet saw their cholesterol levels fall by 12 percent. In an Australian study, a diet rich in barley lowered mildly elevated cholesterol levels in twenty-one men, bringing LDL cholesterol down by 7 percent.

23. RED BEET

Beets are one of the most delicious root vegetables around. Most people have only had the canned variety, which doesn't hold a candle to a freshly pulled beet baked in the oven. These richly colored vegetables are an excellent source of fiber and contain 312 mg of potassium per three-ounce serving. They are also a good source of calcium, phosphorus, and beta-carotene. The leafy greens that sprout from the top of each beet are highly nutritious as well; if you eat beets, steam or stir-fry the greens with garlic, olive oil, or butter.

24. WHEAT GERM AND SPROUTS

If you live in California, you've probably had a shot of wheatgrass juice at some point. This emerald-green elixir is juiced from sprouted wheat, and although its taste leaves some people puckering their lips, it packs a nutrient punch matched by few foods. Fortunately, for those who don't enjoy the taste of fresh wheatgrass juice, freeze-dried wheat sprout powders are available. Sprouted wheat has come a long way since it was first used as a nutritional supplement. Botanists have developed enzyme-rich super sprouts from specially bred wheat, and these sprouts are dried at low temperatures—essential for the preservation of enzyme activity.

Wheat sprouts are incredibly rich in chlorophyll and antioxidant en - zymes, including glutathione peroxidase, catalase, and superoxide dismutase (SOD). All of these antioxidant nutrients are also produced in the body, and the ability to produce enough of them decreases with aging. Wheat sprouts not only introduce more of these nutrients into the body, they also enhance the body's own ability to produce them. Research has shown that life span is proportional to levels of SOD in the heart, brain, and liver; in other words, the more of these antioxidant enzymes you have in your body, the longer you're likely to live. This could have something to do with the ability of SOD to repair damage done to DNA by free radicals or simple wear and tear.

Wheat germ is an integral part of the whole wheat seed that sprouts into wheatgrass. It's a terrific source of insoluble fiber.

25. GINKGO BILOBA

The ginkgo tree has been around for more than 200 million years, and some live for upwards of 4,000 years. This alone is a good testament to the healing powers of this remarkable plant. Chinese herbalists have prescribed ginkgo for the treatment of cough, asthma, and allergic inflammations for more than five millennia. Today, ginkgo is most often touted for its ability to improve circulation, especially throughout the brain and in the legs and feet. It shows promise as a treatment for Alzheimer's disease and other forms of senility, and has been successfully employed as a remedy for vein inflammation (*phlebitis*) and peripheral vascular disease (a common complication of diabetes).

Those who suffer from a chronic ringing in the ears—a condition known as *tinnitus*—have found that ginkgo is one of the only remedies that truly helps them. This is likely due to the improvement of blood flow to the inner ear caused by ginkgo. Substances in the ginkgo plant also act as powerful antioxidants.

Summary of
Green Power Benefits

1. Bilberry

- Improves night vision.
- Strengthens blood vessel walls throughout the body.
- Protects against age-related macular degeneration, glaucoma, and cataracts.
- Protects lungs against toxic pollutants.
- Decreases tendency of blood to clot.
- Protects against stroke.
- Helps relieve allergy symptoms.
- Stimulates enzymes that detoxify carcinogens.

2. Acerola Berry Juice Powder

- Contains 10 times more vitamin C than orange juice.
- Builds tissues.
- Protects against heart disease, vision loss, and cancer.
- Boosts immunity against bacterial and viral infections.
- Protects skin against sun damage.
- Supports health of teeth and bones.
- May extend life span.

3. Astragalus

- Supports body's defensive energy.
- Used in traditional Chinese medicine to treat high blood pressure, heart disease, and diabetes.

- Boosts immune function, especially in cancer patients and children subject to infections.
- Effectively relieves fatigue, loss of appetite, diarrhea, and blood dis - orders.
- May help to prevent the spread of malignant cells into healthy tissues.
- Inhibits the growth of mammary and bladder cancer in animal studies.

4. Spirulina

- Superior source of essential amino acids, fats, vitamins, minerals, and phytonutrients.
- Easily assimilated source of high-quality protein.
- Excellent source of anti-inflammatory omega-6 fat, gamma-linoleic acid.
- Suppresses the growth of *E. coli* and candida yeast.
- Increases immune cell function.
- Rich in chlorophyll, which supports the liver's ability to cleanse the body.
- Anti-inflammatory and antioxidant capability.
- Substances found in spirulina have been shown to be effective against herpes and AIDS viruses, cytomegalovirus, and flu virus.
- Especially protective against mouth cancer.

5. Grape Seed Extract

- Increases body's ability to use and recycle vitamins C and E.
- One of the most potent known antioxidants.
- Protects against Alzheimer's disease.
- Improves strength of capillary walls, which protects against varicose veins, leg swelling, and retinopathy.
- Inhibits LDL oxidation.
- Inhibits excessive blood clotting.
- Improves skin elasticity.
- Helps to heal symptoms of allergy, asthma, and uncontrolled inflammation.
- Antiviral and antibacterial.

- Decreases toxicity of prescription drugs.
- Decreases histamine levels, which helps to treat stress-induced ulcers.

6. Royal Jelly

- Contains full storehouse of B vitamins, which aid in coping with stress.
- Contains full complement of amino acids.
- Rich source of minerals.
- Contains a fatty acid that may be responsible for a queen bee's size and fertility and that may help prevent cancer.
- Increases stamina in athletes.
- Decreases cholesterol levels and excessive blood clotting.
- Speeds healing of skin wounds.
- Contains substances that inhibit bacteria and viruses and may inhibit cancer growth.
- Contains substances that are transformed in the GI tract to natural blood pressure-lowering chemicals.

7. Licorice Root Extract

- Harmonizes other ingredients in traditional Chinese medicine herbal formulas.
- Moisturizes dry mouth.
- Softens, nourishes, coats, lubricates and protects GI tract.
- Natural therapy for ulcers, heartburn, and acid reflux disease.
- Acts as mild adrenal stimulant, increasing energy and soothing inflammation.
- One of the most potent known cancer-protective plants; decreases DNA damage by carcinogens and suppresses growth of cancerous cells.
- Antibacterial and antiviral.
- Has phytoestrogenic qualities that block stronger carcinogenic estrogens.

8. Siberian Ginseng

- Adaptogen that improves endocrine function, stress resistance, and stamina.

- Balances blood sugar levels.
- Improves immune system function against viruses.
- Helps to relieve allergies.
- Improves mental clarity and may help relieve depression.
- Has blood-pressure-normalizing effects.

9. Suma

- Adaptogen that improves endocrine function, stress resistance, and stamina.
- Contains pfaffosides that inhibit tumor growth.
- Contains allantoin, which promotes wound healing.
- Builds immune system function.
- Contains phytosterols that enhance tissue repair.
- May help relieve menopausal and menstrual symptoms, and may improve sexual function.
- Benefits circulatory health and balances cholesterol levels.
- Contains germanium, a rare mineral salt that improves cellular oxygenation.

10. Nova Scotia Dulse

- Good source of trace minerals, especially iodine.
- Supports health of thyroid gland and protects against low thyroid levels.

11. Chlorella

- Contains twice the protein of soybeans and eight times the protein of rice.
- Contains more than twenty vitamins, minerals, and nucleic acids.
- Rich source of anti-inflammatory omega-3 and omega-6 fats.
- Best known source of cleansing, deodorizing, nourishing chlorophyll.
- Highly effective antioxidant.
- Aids detoxification from toxic metals, pesticides, and other chemicals by improving liver function.

- Protects against ill effects of radiation and pollution.
- Improves immune function.
- May protect against cancer growth.
- Detoxifies bowel and relieves bad breath, intestinal gas, and constipation.
- May be an effective ulcer remedy.
- May be an effective remedy for acne, fatigue, asthma, and allergies.
- Can be used before drinking to prevent hangover.
- Fosters improved production of probiotics and vitamin B_{12} in the GI tract.

12. Apple Pectin

- Stabilizes blood sugar.
- Decreases blood cholesterol levels.
- Decreases blood pressure.
- Provides ideal environment for the growth of probiotics in the colon.
- Decreases risk of heart disease.
- Decreases risk of colon cancer.
- Has anti-inflammatory effects on gastrointestinal tract.
- Binds to heavy metals so that they can be flushed out of the body without causing harm.
- Has bacteriostatic effects.

13. Brown Rice Germ

- Cleanses colon and prevents colon cancer.
- Improves bowel regularity.
- Improves elimination of toxins, used-up hormones, and putrefactive bacteria.
- Contains phenols that inhibit growth of human breast and colon cancer cells.
- Oils in rice germ may decrease high cholesterol levels.

14. Green Tea Extract

- Neutralizes free radicals 200 times better than vitamin E.

- Has demonstrated anticancer effects.
- Prevents LDL oxidation.
- Inhibits inflammatory diseases such as rheumatoid arthritis and multiple sclerosis.
- Contains theanine, which enhances effects of cancer medication and decreases their side effects.
- Has antiviral and antibacterial effects.
- Improves digestion.
- Protects against gum disease by killing bacteria and preventing plaque buildup.

15. Bran

- Excellent source of soluble fiber.
- Has been shown to shrink colon polyps.
- Improves action of enzymes that rid the body of carcinogenic chemicals.
- May decrease excessive estrogen levels in premenopausal women, protecting them against cancer.
- Increases satiety and may promote weight loss.

16. Sprouted Barley Malt

- Relieves constipation.
- Relieves symptoms of irritable bowel symptoms and diverticulosis.
- Aids in maintenance of blood sugar balance.

17. Natural Chlorophyll

- Cleanses and deodorizes the GI tract.
- Excellent remedy for bad breath.
- Effective blood builder, especially during pregnancy.
- Helps to eliminate toxins by improving liver function.
- Good source of vitamins, minerals, and trace elements.
- May help to cure kidney stones and upper respiratory infections.

18. Dairy-Free Probiotic Culture

- Improves digestibility of milk and overall digestion.

- Controls toxin-producing putrefactive bacteria.
- Manufactures B vitamins in the GI tract.
- Protects against vaginal yeast and trichomonas infections.
- Improves assimilation of foods.
- Inhibits tumor growth and detoxifies carcinogens.
- Enhances immunity.
- Helps to remedy constipation, diarrhea, and food poisoning.

19. Milk Thistle

- Natural remedy for cirrhosis, fatty liver, and hepatitis.
- Supports liver in day-to-day function.
- Contains silymarin, which has antioxidant power many times of that of vitamin E.
- Protects the liver against free radicals.
- Boosts antioxidant enzyme levels.
- Improves liver cell regeneration 400 to 500 percent.
- Decreases harmful inflammation.
- Contains silibinin, which decreases cancer cell growth.

20. Echinacea

- Increases ability of white blood cells to engulf and destroy pathogens.
- Improves ability of immune cells to "zap" pathogens with the super-oxide anion.
- Shown in clinical studies to shorten duration and severity of colds and flus.
- Inhibits hyaluronidase enzyme, which eats away at healthy cells' natural barriers against pathogens.

21. Alfalfa

- Excellent source of vitamin K, which supports healthy blood clotting, prevents hemorrhage, and aids in calcium retention.
- Cuts levels of harmful LDL cholesterol.

22. Barley

- Good source of soluble fiber.
- Decreased LDL by 7 to 12 percent in men with mildly elevated levels.

23. Red Beet

- Rich in fiber.
- Good source of potassium and calcium.
- Good source of beta-carotene.

24. Wheat Germ and Sprouts

- Rich in chlorophyll.
- Rich in antioxidant enzymes glutathione peroxidase, catalase, and superoxide dismutase.
- May improve body's ability to repair damage and lengthen life span.
- Good source of liver enzymes and soluble and insoluble fiber.

25. Ginkgo Biloba

- Historically used to treat cough, asthma, and allergic inflammation.
- Improves circulation, especially to the brain and lower extremities.
- Promising therapy for Alzheimer's disease and senility.
- Helps to heal phlebitis and peripheral vascular disease.
- One of the only known treatments for tinnitus.

References

Agarwal R, "Cell signaling and regulators of cell cycle as molecular targets for prostate cancer prevention by dietary agents." *Biochem Parmacol* 60 (8) (Oct 15 2000):1051–9.

Amer MA, Lammending AM. "Health maintenance benefits of cultured dairy products." *Cultured Diary Products Journal* 18(1983):16–19.

Anderson JW. *Plant Fiber in Foods.* Lexington, KY: HCF Nutrition Research Foundation, 1990.

Anderson JW., NH Gilinsky, DA Deakins, et al. "Lipid responses of hypercholesterolemic men to oat bran and wheat bran intake." *Am J Clin Nutr* 54(1991):678–683.

Arletti R, A Benelli, A Cavazzuti, et al. "Stimulating property of Turnera diffuse and Pfaffia paniculata extracts on the sexual-behavior of male rats." *Psychopharmacology* (Berl) 140(1) (Mar 1999):15–9.

Ayehunie S, A Belay, TW Baba, et al. "Inhibition of HIV-1 replication by an aqueous extract of Spirulina platensis (Arthrospira platenis)." J Acquir Immune Defic Syndr Hum Retrovirol 18(1)(May 1 1998):7–12 Babu M, et al. "Evaluation of Chemoprevention of Oral Cancer with Spirulin fusitormis." *Nutrition and Cancer* 24(2)(1995): 197–202.

Baojiang G, et al. "Study on Effect and Mechanism of Polysaccharides of Spirulin platenis on Body Immune Functions Improvement." Second Asia-Pacific Conference on Algal Biotechnology (April 25–27, 1994) 24.

Barrett B, M Vohmann, C Calabrese. "Echinacea for upper respiratory infection." *J Fam Pract* 48(8)(Aug 1999):628–35.

Belray A, et al. "Current Knowledge on Potential Health Benefits of Spirulina." *Journal of Applied Phycology* 5(1993):235–41.

Bhat VB, KM Madyastha. "C-phycocyanin: a potent peroxyl radical scavenger in vivo and in vitro." *Biochem Biophys Res Commun* 275(1)(Aug 18 2000):20–5.

Bhat VB, KM Madyastha. "Scavenging of peroxynitrite by phycocyanin and phycocyanobilin from Spriulina platenis: protection against oxidative damage to DNA." *Biochem Biophys Res Commun* 285(2)(Jul 13 2001):262–6.

Bhatia N, J Zhao, DM Wolf. "Inhibition of human carcinoma cell growth and DNA synthesis by silibinin, an active constituent of milk thistle: comparison with silymarin." *Cancer Lett* 147(1-2) (Dec 1 1999):77–84.

Blinkova LP, OB Gorobets, AP Baturo. "Biological activity of Spirulina." *Zh Mikrobiol Epidemiol Immunobiol* 2(Mar-Apr 2001):114–18.

Bomser J, DL Madhavi, K Singletary et al. "In vitro anticancer activity of fruit extracts from Vaccinium species, *Planta Med* 62(3)(Jun1996):212–6.

Buttram HE. "Overuse of antibiotics and the need for alternative." *Townsend Letter* 100 (1991):867–72.

Cara L, C Dubois, P Borel, et al. "Effects of oat bran, rice bran, wheat fiber, and wheat germ on postprandial lipemia in healthy adults." *Am J Clin Nutr* 55(1)(Jan 1992):81–88.

Cho YT. "Studies on Royal Jelly and abnormal cholesterol and triglycerides." *Am Bee J* 117 (1977):36–39.

Clement ML, MM Levine, PA Ristaino, et al. "Exogenous lactobacilli fed to man: their fate and ability to prevent diarrheal disease." *Prog Food Nutr* 7(3-4)(1983):29–37.

Craig W, L Beck. "Phytochemicals: health protective effects." *Can J Diet Pract Res* 60(2)(Summer 1999):78–84.

Das DK, M Sato, PS Ray, et al. "Cardioprotection of red wine: role of polyphenolica antioxidants." *Drugs Exp Clin Res* 25(2-3)(1999):115–20.

Davydov M, AD Krikorian. "Eleutherococcus senticosus (Rupr. & Maxim.) Maxim. (Araliaceae) as an adaptogen: a closer look." *J Ethnopharmacol* 72(3)(Oct 2000):345–93.

DeOliveira F. "Pfaffia paniculata (Martius) Kuntze—Brazilian ginseng." *Rev Bras Farmacog* 1(1)(1986):86–92.

Deyama T, S Nishibe, Y Nakazawa. "Constituents and pharmacological effects of Eucommia and Siberian ginseng." *Acta Pharmacol Sin* 222(12)(Dec 2001):1057–70.

Fine AM. "Oligomeric proanthocyanidin complexes: history, structure, and phytopharmaceutical applications." *Altern Med Rev* 5(2)(Apr 2000):144–51.

Fujiwara S, J Imai, M Fujiwara, et al. "A potent antibacterial protein in royal jelly. Purification and determination of the primary structure of royalism." *J Biol Chem* 265(19)(Jul 5 1990):11333–37.

Giles JT, CT Palat 3rd, SH Chien, et al. "Evaluation of echinacea for the treatment of the common cold." *Pharmacotherapy* 20(6)(Jun 2000):690–7.

Glattharr-Saalmuller B, F Sacher, A Esperester. "Antiviral activity of an extract derived from roots of Eleutherococcus senticosus." *Antiviral Res* 50(3)(Jun 2001):223–8.

Goldin BR, SL Gorbach. "The effect of milk and *Lactobacillus* feeding on human intestinal bacterial enzyme activity." *Am J Clin Nutr* 39(1984):756–61.

Gorbach SL. "Lactic acid bacteria and human health." *Annals of Medicine* 22(1990):37–41.

Gorban EM, et al. "Clinical and experimental study of spirulina efficacy in chronic diffuse liver disease." *Lik Sprava* 6(Sep 2000):89–93.

Guzman S, A Gato, JM Calleja. "Anti-inflammatory, analgesic and free radical scavenging activities of the marine microalgae Chlorella Stigmatophora and Phaeodactylum tricornutum." *Phytother Res* 15(3)(May 2001):224–30.

Hamilton-Miller JM. "Anti-carcinogenic properties of tea (Camellia sinensis)." *J Med Microbial* 50(4)(Apr 2001):299–302.

Hayashi K, et al. "An Extract from Spirulina platensis is a Selective Inhibitor of Herpes Simplex Virus Type I Penetration into HeLa Cells." *Phytotherapy Research* 7(1993):76–80.

Hayashi O, et al. "Enhancement of antibody production in mice by dietary Spirulina platensis." *Journal of Nutritional Sciences and Vitaminology* 40(1994):431–441.

Head KA, "Natural therapies for ocular disorders, part two: cataracts and glaucoma," *Altern Med Rev* 6(2)(Apr 2001):141–66.

Helsby NA, S Zhu, AE Pearson, et al. "Antimutagenic effects of wheat bran diet through modification of xenobiotic metabolizing enzymes." *Mutat Res* 454(1-2)(Nov 6 2000):77–88.

Hosono A, T Kasina, T Kada, et al. "Anti-mutagenic properties of lactic-acid-cultured milk on chemical and fecal mutagens." *J Dairy Sci* 69(1986):2237–42.

Hudson EA, PA Dinh, T Kokubun, et al. "Characterization of potentially chemopreventive phenols in extracts of brown rice that inhibits the growth of human breast and colon cancer cells." *Cancer Epidemiol Biomarkers Prev* 9(11)(Nov 2000):1163–70.

Jeong HJ, HN Koon, NI Myung, et al. "Inhibitory effects of mast cell-mediated allergic reactions by cell cultured Siberian Ginseng." *Immunopharmacol Immunotoxicol* 23(1)(Feb 2001): 107–17.

Jiao Y, J Wen, X Yu. "Influence of flavonoid of Astragalus membranaceus' stem and leaves on the function of cell mediated immunity in mice." *Zhongguo Zhong Xi Yi Jie He Za Zhi* 19(6)(Jun 1999):356–8.

Joshi SS, CA Kuszynski, D Bagchi. "The cellular and molecular basis of health benefits of grape seed proanthocyanidin extract." *Curr Pharm Biotechnol* 2(2)(Jun 2001): 187–200.

Jung YD, LM Ellis. "Inhibition of tumor invasion and angiogenesis by epigallocatechin gallate (EGCG), a major component of green tea." *Int J Exp Pathol* 81(6)(Dec 2001):309–16.

Katiyar SK, CA Elmets. "Green tea polyphenolic antioxidants and skin photoprotection (Review)." *Int J Oncol* 18(6)(Jun 2001):1307–13.

Kimura Y, C Miyagi, M Kimura, et al. "Structural features of N-glycans linked to royal jelly glycoproteins: structures of high-mannose type, hybrid type, and biantennary type glycans." *Biosci Biotechnol Biochem* 64(10)(Oct 2000):2109–20.

Kimura Y, N Washino, and M Yonekura. "N-linked sugar chains of 350-kDa royal jelly glyco-protein." *Biosci Biotechnol Biochem* 59(3)(Mar 1995):507–9.

Kurachige S, Y Akuzawa, F Endo. "Effects of astragali radix extract on carcinogenesis, cyto-kine production, and cytotoxicity in mice treated with a carcinogen, N-butyl-N'-butanolni-trosamine." *Cancer Invest* 17(1)(1999):30–5.

Lin CC, YP Lu, YR Lu, et al. "Inhibition by dietary dibenzoylmethane of mammary gland proliferation, formation of DMBA-DNA adducts in mammary glands, and mammary tumorigenesis in Sencar mice." *Cancer Lett* 168(2)(Jul 2001):125–32.

Logan AC, C Wong. "Chronic fatigue syndrome: Oxidative stress and dietary modifications." *Altern Med Rev* 6(5)(Oct 2001):450–9.

Lorenzani, Shirley S, Ph.D. *Dietary Fiber: Its Surprising Range of Therapeutic and Protective Health Benefits.* New Canaan, CT: Keats Publishing, Inc.,1988.

Ma J, NY Fu, DB Pang, et al. "Apoptosis induced by isoliquiritigenin in human gastric cancer MGC-803 cells." *Planta Med* 67(8)(Nov 2001):754–7.

Majeed, Muhammed, Ph.D., and Lakshmi Prakash, Ph.D. *Lactospore: The Effective Probiotic.* Piscataway, NJ:NutriScience Publishers, Inc., 1998.

Martinez A, I Cambero, Y Ikken, et al. "Protective Effect of Broccoli, Onion, Carrot, and Licorice Extracts against Cytotoxicity of N-Nitrosamines Evaluated by 3-(4,5-Dimethylthia-zol-s-yl)-2,5-diphenyltetrazolium Bromide Assay." *J Agric Food Chem* 46(2)(Feb 16 1998): 585-9.

Matsui T, A Yukiyoshi, S. Doi, et al. "Gastrointestinal enzyme production of bioactive pep-tides from royal jelly protein and their antihypertensive ability in SHR." *J Nutr Biochem* 13(2)(Feb 2002):80–86.

Mindell, Earl L., R.Ph., Ph.D., and Donald R Yance, Jr. C.N., M.H. *Dr. Earl Mindell's Russian Energy Secret.* North Bergen, NJ: Basic Health Publications, Inc., 2001.

Mindell, Earl L., R.Ph., Ph.D., with Virginia L Hopkins. *Dr. Earl Mindell's What You Should Know About Fiber and Digestion.* New Canaan, CT: Keats Publishing, Inc., 1997.

Mitsuoka T. "Intestinal flora and host." *Asian Medical Journal* 37(7)(1988):400–9.

Mohan JC, R Arora, M Khalilullah, et al. "Preliminary observations on effect of *L. sporogenes* on serum lipid levels in hypercholesterolemic patients." *Indian J Med Res* 92(1990):431–42.

Molgaard J, H von Schenck, and AG Ollson. "Alfalfa seeds lower low density lipoproteins cholesterol and apolipoprotein B concentrations in patients with type II hyperlipoproteinemia." *Atherosclerosis* 65(1-2)(May 1987):173–9.

Nagasawa H, K Watanabe, M Yoshida, et al. "Effects of gold banded lily (Lilium auratum Lindl) or Chinese milk vetch (Astragalus sinicus L) on spontaneous mammary tumorigenesis in SHN mice," *Atnticancer Res* 4A(Jul-Aug 2001):2323–8.

No author listed. "Silybum marianum (mild thistle)." *Altern Med Rev* (Aug 4 1999);(4):272-4.

Ohno K, S Narushima, S Takeuchi, et al. "Inhibitory effect of apple pectin and culture condensate of Bifidobacterium longum on colorectal tumors induced by 1,2-dimethylhydrazine in transgenic mice harboring human prototype c-Ha-ras genes." *Exp Anim* 49(4)(Oct 2000): 305–7.

Oka H, Y Emori, N Kobayashi, et al. "Suppression of allergic reactions by royal jelly in association with restoration of macrophage function and the improvement of Th1/Th2 cell responses." *Int Immunopharmacol* 1(3)(Mar 2001):521–32.

Otles S, R Pire. "Fatty acid composition of Chlorella and Spirulina microalgae species." *JAOAC Int* 84(6)(Nov-Dec 2002):1708–14.

Percival SS., "Use of Echinacea in medicine." *Biochem Pharmacol* 60(2)(Jul 2000):155–8.

Pinero Estrada JE, P Bermejo Bescos, AM Villar del Fresno. "Antioxidant activity of different fractions of Spirulina platensis protean extract." *Farmaco* 56(5-7)(May-Jul 2001):497–500.

Pirich C, P Schmid, J Pidlich, et al. "Lowering cholesterol with Anticholest—a high fiber guar-apple pectin drink." *Wien Klin Wochenschr* 104(11)(1992):314–6.

Potievskii EG, Sh Shavakhabov, VM Bondarenko, et al. "Experimental and clinical studies of the effect of pectin on the causative agents of acute intestinal infections." *Zh Mikrobiol Epidemiol Immunobiol* Suppl 1(Aug-Sep 1994):106–9.

Premkumar K, A Pachiappan, SK Abraham, et al. "Effect of Spirulina fusiformis on cyclophosphamide and mitomycin-C induced gentoxicity and oxidative stress in mice." *Fitoterapia* 72(8)(Dec 2001):906–11.

Preuss HG, D Wallerstedt, N Talpur, et al. "Effect of niacin-bound chromium and grape seed proanthocyanidin extract on the lipid profile of hypercholesterolemic subjects: a pilot study." *J Med* 31(5-6)(2000):227–46.

Pugh N, SA Ross, HN ElSohly, et al. "Isolation of three high molecular weight polysaccharide preparations with potent immunostimulatory activity from Spirulina platensis, aphanizomenon flosaquae and Chlorella pyrenoidosa." *Planta Med* 67(8)(Nov 2001):737–42.

Quan J, G Du. "Protective effect of Astragalus membranaceus (Fisch.) Bge. and Hedysarym polybotrys Hand.–Mass. on experimental model of cerebral ischemia in rats." *Zhongguo Zhong Xi Yi Jie He Za Zhi* 23(6)(Jun 1998):371–3.

Rafi MM, BC Vastano, N Zhu, et al. "Novel Polyphenol Molecule Isolated from Licorice Root (Glycrrhiza glabra) Induces Apoptosis, G2/M Cell Cycle Arrest, and Bcl-2 Phosphorylation in Tumor Cell Lines." *J Agric Food Chem* 50(4)(Feb 2002):677–84.

Ray SD, D Patel, V Wong, et al. "In vivo protection of DNA damage associated apoptotic and necrotic cell deaths during acetaminophen-induced nephrotoxicity, amiodarone-induced lung toxicity and doxorubicin-induced cardiotoxicity by a novel IH636 grape seed proanthocyanidin extract." *Res Commun Mol Pathol Pharmacol* 107(1-2)(2000):137–66.

Reddy CM, VB Bhat, G Kiranmei, et al. "Selective inhibition of cyclooxygenase-2 by C-phycocyanin, a biliprotein from Spirulina platensis." *Biochem Biophys Res Commun* 277(2)(Nov 2000):599–603.

Reddy BS, Y Hirose, LA Cohen, et al. "Preventive potential of wheat bran fractions against experimental colon carcinogenesis: implications for human colon cancer prevention." *Cancer Res* 60(17)(Sep 2000):4792–7.

Reddy BS. "Prevention of colon carcinogenesis by components of dietary fiber." *Anticancer Res* 19(5A)(Sep-Oct 1999):3681–3.

Rodriguez-Hernandez A, JL Ble-Castillo, MA Juarez-Orapena, et al. "Spirulina maxima prevents fatty liver formation in CD-1 male and female mice with experimental diabetes." *Life Sci* 69(9)(Jul 2001):1029–37.

Romay C, N Ledon, R Gonzalez. "Effects of phycocyanin extract on prostaglandin e2 levels in mouse ear inflammation test." *Arzneimittelforschung* 50(12)(Dec 2000):1106–9.

Rountree, Bob, M.D., and Carol Colman. *Immunotics: A Revolutionary Way to Fight Infection, Beat Chronic Illness, and Stay Well.* New York, NY: G. P. Putnam's Sons, 2000.

Roychowdhury S, G Wolf, G Keilhoff, et al. "Protection of primary glial cells by grape seed proanthocyanidin extract against nitrosative/oxidative stress." *Nitric Oxide* 5(2)(2001): 137–49.

Saikatsu S, K Ikeno, Y Hanada, et al. "Physiologically active substances in the oral excreta produced by honey bee—effects of royal jelly on silkworm." *Ou Daigaku Shigakushi* 16(3)(Nov 1989):113–6.

Saller R, R Meier, R Brignoli. "The use of silymarin in the treatment of liver diseases." *Drugs* 61(14)(2001):2035–63.

Schulten B, M Bulitta, B Ballering-Bruhl, et al. "Efficacy of Echinacea purpurea in patients with a common cold. A placebo-controlled, randomized, double-blind clinical test." *Arzneimittelforshung* 51(7)(2001):563–8.

Sen CK, D Bagchi. "Regulation of inducible adhesion molecule expression in human endothelial cells by grape seed proanthocyanidin extract." *Mol Cell Biochem* 216(1-2)(Jan 2001):1–7.

Sengupta S, JJ Tjandra, PR Gibson. "Dietary fiber and colorectal neoplasia." *Dis Colon Rectum* 44(7)(Jul 2001):1016–33.

Shahani KM, AD Ayebo. "Role of dietary Lactobacilli in gastrointestinal micro ecology." *Am J Clin Nutr* 33(1980):2448–457.

Shahani KM, et al. "Antitumor activity of fermented colostrums and milk." *J Food Protect* 46(1983):385–6.

Shamsuddin AM, I Vucenik. "Mammary tumor inhibition by IP6: a review." *Anticancer Res* (5A)(Sep-Oct 1999):3671–4.

Smith-Barbaro P, D Hanson D, BS Reddy. "Carcinogen binding to various types of dietary fiber." *J Natl Cancer Inst* 67(2)(Aug 1981):495–7.

Steenblock, David, B.S., M.Sc., D.O. *Chlorella: Natural Medicinal Algae*. Mission Viejo, CA: Aging Research Institute, 1996.

Sueoka N, et al. "A new function of green tea: prevention of lifestyle-related diseases." *Ann N Y Acad Sci* 918(Apr 2001):274–80.

Sugano M, K Koba, E Tsuji. "Health benefits of rice bran oil." *Anticancer Res* 19(5A)(Sep-Oct 1999):3651–7.

Sver L, N Orsolic, Z Tadic, et al. "A royal jelly as a new potential immunomodulator in rats and mice." *Comp Immunol Microbiol Infect Dis* 19(1)(Jan 1996):31–8.

Tamir S, M Eizenberg, D Somjen, et al. "Estrogen-like activity of glabrene and other constituents isolated from licorice root." *J Steroid Biochem Mol Biol* 78(3)(Sep 2001):291–8.

Tanaka Y, H Kikuzaki, S Fukada, et al. "Antibacterial compounds of licorice against upper airway respiratory tract pathogens." *J Nutr Si Vitaminol* (Tokyo) 47(3)(Jun 2001):270–3.

Tazawa K, K Yatuzuka, M Yatuzuka, et al. "Dietary fiber inhibits the incidence of hepatic metastasis with the anti-oxidant activity and portal scavenging functions." *Hum Cell* 12(4) (Dec 1999):189–96.

Tazawa K, H Okami, I Yamashita, et al. "Anticarcinogenic action of apple pectin on fecal enzyme activities and mucosal or portal prostaglandin E2 levels in experimental rat colon carcinogenesis." *J Exp Clin Cancer Res* 16(1)(Mar 1997):33–8.

Thakur BR, RK Singh, AK Handa. "Chemistry and uses of pectin—a review." *Crit Rev Food Sci Nutr* 37(1)(Feb 1997):47–73.

Tosetti F, N Ferrari, S De Flora, et al. "Angioprevention: angiogenesis is a common and key target for cancer chemopreventive agents." *FASEB J* 16(1)(Jan 1992):2–14.

Upsani CD, A Khera, R Balaraman. "Effect of lead with vitamin E, C, or Spirulina on malondialdehyde, conjugated dienes and hydroperoxides in rats." *Indian J Exp Biol* 39(1)(Jan 2001):70–4.

Wang D, C Wang C, Y Tian. "Effect of total flavonoids of Astraglus on nitroxide in ischemia reperfusion injury." *Zhongguo Zhong Xi Yi Jie He Za Zhi* 19(4)(Apr 1999):221–3.

Wang ZY, DW Nixon. "Licorice and cancer." *Nutr Cancer* 39(1)(2001):1–11.

Watanabe T, M Watanabe, Y Watanabe, et al. "Effects of oral administration of Pfaffia paniculata (Brazilian ginseng) on incidence of spontaneous leukemia in AKR/J mice." *Cancer Detect Prev* 24(2)(2000):173–8.

Weisburger JH. "Tea and health: the underlying mechanisms." *Proc Soc Exp Biol Med* 220(4) (Apr 1999):271–5.

Yang CS, JY Chung, GY Yang, et al. "Mechanisms of inhibition of carcinogenesis by tea." *Biofactors* 13(1-4)(2000):73–9.

Zhang HQ, AP Lin, Y Sun, et al. "Chemo- and radio-protective effects of polysaccharide of Spirulina platensis on hemopoetic system of mice and dogs." *Acta Pharmacol Sin* 22(12)(Dec 2001):1121–4.

Index

About the Authors

Earl Mindell, R.Ph., Ph.D.

Earl Mindell, R.Ph., Ph.D., is a professor of nutrition at Pacific Western University. In addition to writing several hundred articles on the subject of alternative health, Dr. Mindell has written more than thirty books and booklets, including the bestselling *Earl Mindell's Vitamin Bible* and *Earl Mindell's Herb Bible.* Dr. Mindell received his pharmacy degree from North Dakota State University and his doctorate in nutrition from Pacific Western University.

Tony O'Donnell

Tony O'Donnell is a health advocate who appears on network television regularly and has his own radio show in Phoenix, Arizona. *Greens Are Good for You* is his second book. His initial publication, *Miracle Super Foods That Heal,* was published in 1998, reprinted in 2001, and reprinted for a second time in 2002. He was awarded the 2001 Man of the Year by the Leukemia Society of Phoenix, Arizona.

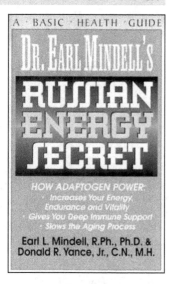